W9-APM-236

Yoga For Beginners: Essential Poses For Yoga Beginners

Become A Yoga Expert With The Best Yoga Poses For Flexibility

By: Amy Gilchrist

ISBN-13: 978-1490345482

TABLE OF CONTENTS

Amy Gilchrist

PUBLISHERS NOTES

Disclaimer

This publication is intended to provide helpful and informative material. It is not intended to diagnose, treat, cure, or prevent any health problem or condition, nor is intended to replace the advice of a physician. No action should be taken solely on the contents of this book. Always consult your physician or qualified health-care professional on any matters regarding your health and before adopting any suggestions in this book or drawing inferences from it.

The author and publisher specifically disclaim all responsibility for any liability, loss or risk, personal or otherwise, which is incurred as a consequence, directly or indirectly, from the use or application of any contents of this book.

Any and all product names referenced within this book are the trademarks of their respective owners. None of these owners have sponsored, authorized, endorsed, or approved this book.

Always read all information provided by the manufacturers' product labels before using their products. The author and publisher are not responsible for claims made by manufacturers.

Paperback Edition 2013

Manufactured in the United States of America

Amy Gilchrist

DEDICATION

This book is dedicated to Shakira, my doting yoga instructor.

CHAPTER 1- INTRODUCTION TO BASIC YOGA

The elementary techniques associated with yoga go back more than five thousand years. Back then the main purpose was to achieve a better understanding of self, long life and health as well as personal freedom and this gave birth to a process which made use of mental and physical exercise which has become a worldwide phenomenon over the years. Yoga means to yoke together or join and it joins the mind and body.

Yoga is founded on three principles, meditation, breathing and exercise. The exercises are meant to augment overall health and efficiency by placing pressure on the glandular systems of the body. The body is viewed as the main tool that enables an individual to evolve and work and it must be cared for and treated with respect.

The techniques for breathing are founded on the premise that in the body, the source of life is breath. A student that is learning the techniques of yoga will gradually increase the control in breathing to improve the way the mind and body functions.

These two forms of breathing and exercise then make the body ready for meditation and the student will find it easier to quiet the mind and get rid of the stress that was built up during the course of the day. Regular practice of yoga will produce a body that is capable and strong and a mind that is bright and clear. The following chapters outline thirty one basic yoga poses along with illustrations.

CHAPTER 2- STANDING SIDEWAYS BENDING ONE ARM- KONASANA

To Do Standing Sideways Bending One Arm - Konasana follow these steps:

Stand up tall with arms at the sides and center your mind for a few seconds. Open your feet in a wide stance. Your legs should form an upside-down "V" on the floor. Keep your back straight. Turn the right foot to the side at 90 degrees from the body. Move the left foot slightly outward to steady the pose.

Inhale and slowly bring both arms out in a straight, 180-degree line from the shoulders. Hold the arms out straight and maintain an elongated back.

Exhale. Bend your body to the right by bending your right knee. The left arm maintains its straight position from the shoulder, but it is now pointing upwards. The right knee does not go past the right toes.

Place the area below your right elbow against your right thigh. Look up at your left hand. As you bend to the right, gently stretch the left hip muscles. Feel your body lengthening. There should be an invisible straight line from the tips of the skyward fingers down to the right foot.

Hold for 30 seconds and arise. Repeat by bending the left leg and stretching the other side of the body. A variation is shown below

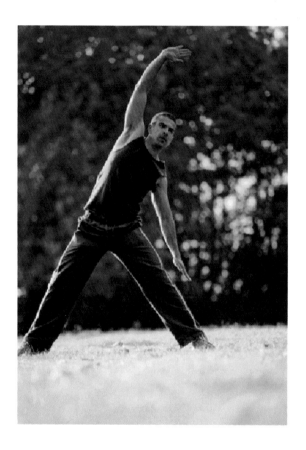

Chapter 3- Sideways Bending Using

Both Arms- Konasana 2

Create a comfortable exercise space that maximizes safety during your routine and then follow these directions to do this exercise properly. This is a relaxing exercise but as always, will challenge someone that is just beginning a routine. Do not perform this exercise unless you are cleared to do so by a doctor. If you've been cleared to perform this exercise, or are in very good health, then you will find that this is an extremely relaxing exercise to perform.

Begin standing with your feet approximately 2 feet apart. Raise arms overhead and join your hands together, placing palms flat together. Fold fingers to form a triangle position (Breathe in).

Take a breath out while bending to your right. Keep elbows straight and press feet to the ground while moving your hips to the left. HOLD this position, feeling a stretch, and then slowly relaxing into the position. Continue to breathe gently. Return to a standing position. Repeat

Repeat this as many times as you are comfortable or have worked out for your routine. While it is important to challenge yourself, it is also important to build into an exercise routine comfortably, without undue stress that might cause health problems. As always, make sure that you are healthy enough to perform this exercise.

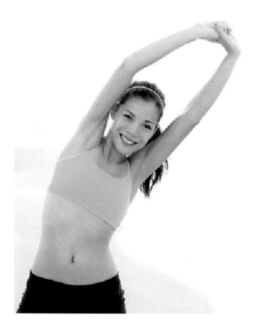

CHAPTER 4- STANDING SPINAL TWIST-KATICHAKRASANA

The spinal twist is a yoga posture that takes little time to maneuver. The name, Katichakrasana, literally breaks down in translation to "turning the waist like a wheel." It helps keep the back muscles about the waist area flexible and strong.

To perform the spinal twist one must first stand with your feet together. Legs must be together but relaxed; do not lock the knees. The arms are then outstretched directly in front and parallel to the ground. The palms should face each other, almost as if an item was being held in the outstretched arms. The spacing of the arms should be about shoulder width apart. Remember to keep the shoulder at a neutral posture and not hunched-up into the neck.

At the same time as exhaling, twist to the right. As you are doing this, turn the head as if to look over the right shoulder. Be sure to keep the arms parallel to the ground and spaced as if you were holding a package in your outstretched arms. Keeping your feet flat on the ground enhances the stretch you will feel.

Return to center as you inhale. The stretch is repeated to the left in the same manner with another exhale. You will really feel the stretch in your lower back. Inhale and once again return to center. A variation is shown below.

Yoga For Beginners

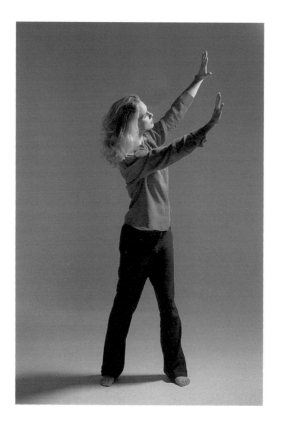

CHAPTER 5- STANDING FORWARD BEND- HASTAPADASANA

Begin by standing on your mat with your feet together, arms by your sides. Raise your arms straight above your head, stretching your fingertips to the ceiling. Maintaining a flat back, begin to bend forward from the hip, keeping your upper arms by your ears as you bring your arms and torso down at the same time, stretching your fingers forward. Follow this motion, keeping your knees locked, until you are reaching towards the ground.

Imagine the ideal form in which you are bent almost completely in half. Depending on your level of flexibility, either put your hands on the floor, underneath your feet, or somewhere on your legs, as far down as you can reach while keeping your legs completely straight.

Never bend your knees or you will lose the stretch. With your hands in place, tuck your head in and stretch, aiming to use your hands to pull the top of your head down towards the ground, and your nose in towards your knees. You should feel an intense stretching sensation. However, if the pressure in your hamstrings or knees becomes too intense, do not bend your knees, but relax and allow your hands and upper body to rise upwards only a few inches until you are ready to stretch again. Maintain this stretch for at least 30 seconds.

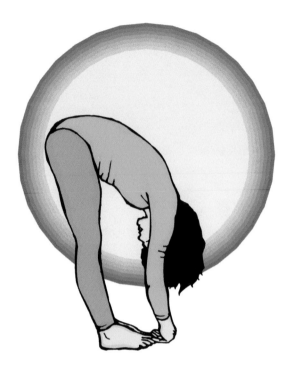

CHAPTER 6- STANDING BACKWARD BEND-ARDHA CHAKRASANA

Begin by standing on your mat with your feet slightly apart, your arms by your sides. Raise your hands and press them together in front of your chest with the palms touching. Interlace your fingers and fold them down so that only your index fingers are pointing to the ceiling. Keeping your palms pressed together, stretch your arms upwards so that your upper arms are next to your ears, and look up. Keep your fingers pointed and your arms straight as you slowly begin to push your arms back. Let your head follow in line with your fingers so that your back begins to bend. Go slowly; this may be difficult for the beginner.

Allow your chest to open up. Continue to breathe as you stretch your arms back, imagining that you are trying to touch the wall behind you with your pointed fingers. Always keep your head in line by looking for your hands and keeping your ears roughly parallel with your biceps. Some advanced yogis will begin to see the floor as they bend over backwards. When you reach the full extent of your stretch, hold yourself in that position, being sure to continue to breathe and listen to your body so as not to stress your back. Slowly reverse the process and begin to come back up, finishing with your hands in front of your chest.

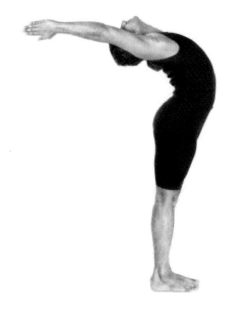

CHAPTER 7- TRIANGLE POSE- TRIKONASANA

Traditionally, the Trikonasana begins in a standing pose with feet together, spine straight, and hands clasped on the chest in the namaste gesture. The practitioner then lowers their arms down to the side of their body and jumps their feet about three feet apart. If you are a beginner, you can slide one foot to the side two or three feet.

The alignment of your feet is going to be important in this pose. To help you create the correct balance, pretend there is a straight line underneath your feet. Twist your left foot into an outward position while turning your right foot inward at a 45 degree angle on this imaginary line. Your torso should remain facing forward with your arms down by your sides.

The next step is to begin the lean sideways. Raise your arms up from your side to shoulder level. Your fingertips should point straight outward to the side. Twist your head to the right and slowly hinge from your hips to the left until your fingers touch your ankle.

To complete the asana you must lift back to the starting position. Begin by pulling your body upright by reaching your right arm outward. Once in an upright position you can bring your feet together and lower your arms back to your sides.

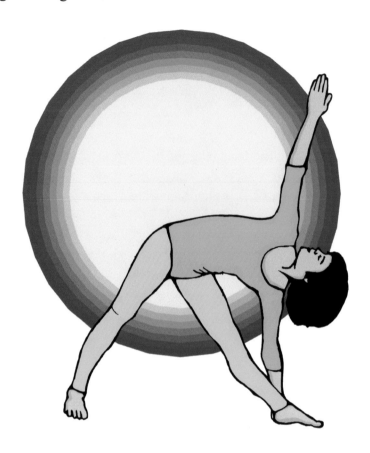

Chapter 8- Warrior Pose- Veerabhadrasana or Virabhadrasana

The warrior pose starts in the mountain pose. Stand straight. Feet should match the width of your hips. Arms should hang down at its sides. Palms of hands should face the body. Let the weight rest on your toes while your left foot turn to the left and right foot turns to the right. Make shoulders relaxed and broad. Hold in your ribs in the belly's direction and move the back of the pelvis from the lower back. Concentrate while breathing in and out. If done correctly breathing patterns should stretch body upwards. Look straight ahead.

After forming the mountain pose jump or move your left leg sideways; when done correctly feet should start to separate further from each other. The left foot must be four feet apart from your right foot. Now turn your left foot 90 degrees to the left. Turn your right foot 45 degrees to the left. Remain in this position while turning your upper body to the left. Now that everything is facing to the left bend the left knee. The left knee is the one with the foot facing 90 degrees. The bended knee should be directly above your foot. Raise your arms in the air. Palms of your hands must face each other in the air while fingers are stretched out.

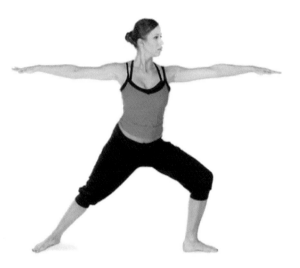

CHAPTER 9- STANDING FORWARD BEND WITH FEET APART- PARSARITA PADOTANASANA

A standing forward bend with feet apart, also known as Parsarita Padotanasana, is a great way to stretch the lower back, inner thighs, and spine. To begin the pose first you will need to stand upright while placing both feet approximately 3 - 4 feet apart. Make sure that you are very well balanced when positioning your feet. Next you will want to take a deep breath and stretch your arms gently over your head. Moving right along, next exhale; gently lean all the way forward at the hip while keeping your spine completely straight. Lastly you will want to place both hands on to the ground directly in front of you, as this will further deepen or extend the stretching.

While you are in the pose you can attempt to move your feet further apart, as this will enhance the stretching of your inner thighs. You should also strongly focus on possessing a firm balance throughout the pose, while maintaining a slow, steady, and rhythmic breathing pattern.

This pose should be practiced two or more times a week. Over time you will notice that it will greatly strengthen your ankles, feet, legs, and abdomen. The pose will also lengthen your spine to a more natural state, as the stretching motion greatly helps to decrease compression between the individual vertebrae.

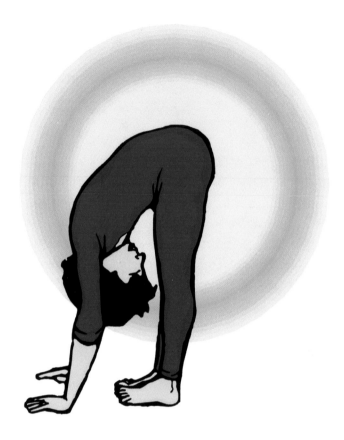

CHAPTER 10- TREE POSE- VRIKSHASANA

First, stand up straight and focus quietly in Mountain Pose (Tadasana).Shift your weight to your left foot until you feel rooted.

Lift the right foot. Place the sole on the inside of the left thigh. Your toes are pointed downward. Your right knee is pointed to the right. Bring both hands to the center of your chest; palms pushed together (Namaste).

Keeping the hands together, bring them over your head. Elbows are to the sides. Hold this position for 30 seconds. With practice, increase the hold up to two minutes to improve balance and strengthen legs.

To release:

Bring the hands down to the sides. Lower the foot slowly to the floor. Stand straight in Tadasana for several breaths. Repeat Vrikshasana lifting left foot.

Some important things to remember: If you cannot bring the foot to the inside of the thigh, then rest the sole further down on the leg where it is comfortable. Avoid pushing the knee out to the side with your foot. At first you may just want to leave the hands in the Namaste position at the chest. It is fine to begin practice by holding onto a chair with one arm or by leaning on a wall.

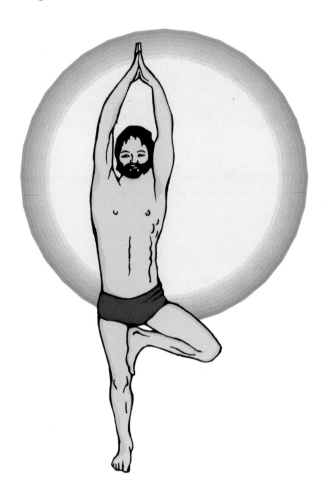

CHAPTER 11- CHAIR POSE- UTKATASANA

To do the chair pose you usually start by standing straight up with your arms hanging by your sides. The toes should be relaxed and spread apart.

While standing erect breathe in then lift your arms up in the air so they are straight over your head. It is a matter of choice if you want to hold your hands apart or join them together.

When you exhale try to imagine you are sitting down in a chair. Bend your knees slowly and gently until your body is posed as if you were sitting in a chair. An objective is to have your thighs as close to parallel with the floor as possible.

It is important to try to keep your back as straight as possible while you are assuming this pose. While assuming the chair pose, breathe in and out several times then return to the standing straight up position.

If you find it difficult to assume this pose at first you can utilize a wall to help you carry it out. Simply place your back a few inches away from a wall and while you are assuming the chair pose you can rest your lower back on the wall. This helps to make it easier to perform the pose by putting less pressure on your thighs.

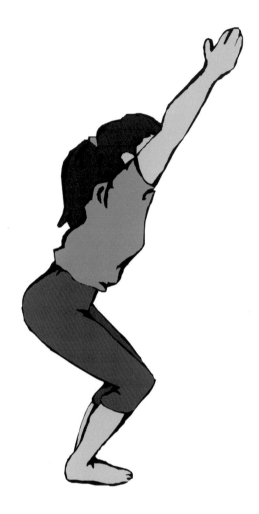

CHAPTER 12- ONE-LEGGED FORWARD BEND- JANU SHIRASASANA

To begin the one-legged forward bend, also known as Janu Shirasasana, you will need to sit upright, stretch your legs out in front of you, all the while keeping your spine completely straight. Next fold your left leg at the knee joint and then gently place your foot against your inner right thigh. For the next step take in a deep breath, lift both arms directly above your head, reach out towards the sky, and then slightly twist towards the right.

Moving along, next exhale deeply and then lean forward at the hip while pointing your chin toward your feet. It is very helpful if you can grasp your toes during this stretch. Once you have attained the position continue to hold it while slowly and deeply breathing. Once done, repeat the stretch using the opposite side of your body.

The benefits of this stretch can greatly increase the health and well being of you lower back, especially the spinal vertebrae. This stretch is highly recommended for anyone who spends long periods of time seated. Another benefit of this stretch is that it gently massages your abdominal organs, which contrary to popular belief can actually be realigned to a much more natural position with regular stretching. Repeat this stretch several times a week to receive its full benefits.

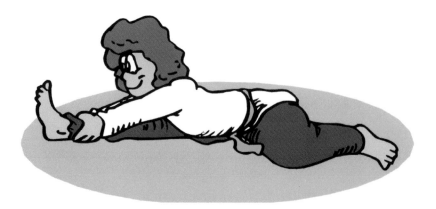

CHAPTER 13- TWO-LEGGED FORWARD BEND- PASCHIMOTTANASANA

Sit on the floor with your legs together. Your back is straight, and the top of your head is reaching for the sky. Hands are palm down on your thighs. Inhale and exhale twice, then slowly slide your hands down your legs.

Grab hold of your feet. If you cannot reach them, grab your ankles or any part of your legs as long as you remain comfortable. Inhale. Then on the exhale, lower your body as far as it will go to the floor. Bend the elbows as needed. The stretch should be felt through the back and hamstrings. Do not overstrain. Hold the pose for 30 seconds.

Inhale and allow the hands to slide up as you come up. Relax your muscles and breathe gently a few times.

This asana can be adapted to meet individual needs by modifying the intensity of the stretch. You can leave the knees bent to avoid over-stretching the hamstrings. Sitting on a folded towel helps push the torso forward. The head can be supported on a block or towel in the lap. A strap placed around the balls of the feet can be used to pull, as long as the shoulders are not tensed.

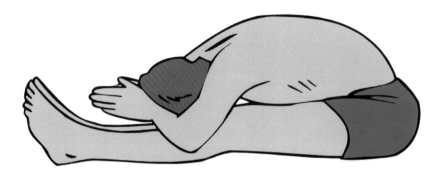

Amy Gilchrist

CHAPTER 14- INCLINED PLANE-POORVOTTANASANA

The inclined plane is a great yoga pose that helps you focus and work on balance. Here's how you can do it and achieve the strength and great flexibility involved with the pose"

Lay on your body in a staff position. Keep your arms behind your hips and have your fingers pointed towards your body as you begin to lean into your palms. When lifting the hips up slowly from the floor, be sure to inhale deep. As the hips are lifting towards the ceiling, use your legs by squeezing your knee caps tight as well as your thighs, that way you get the full range of motion. The bottoms of your feet should be pressed firmly down into the floor and you should squeeze your butt tightly to help with stability and muscle growth. Next, draw your shoulder blades together and lift them through the sternum.

Keep your body aligned straight from toes to shoulders. If you feel comfortable with it, you can drop your head back for an extra stretch and flexibility work. Breathe and hold this last position for 2-6 seconds while taking long, deep breaths. When you are finished, slowly release your hips back to the floor. Do this once or twice daily for complete relaxation and flexibility work in your back and thighs.

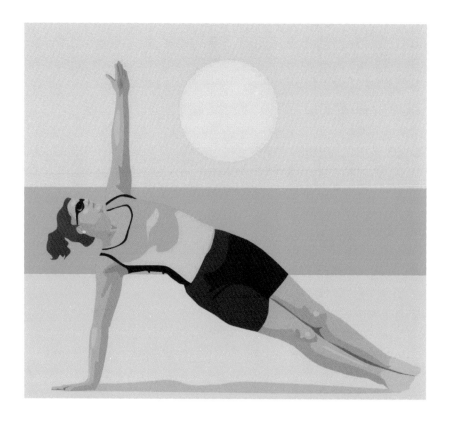

CHAPTER 15- SITTING HALF SPINAL TWIST- ARDHA MATSYENDRASANA

Do the Half Spinal Twist - Ardha Matsyendrasana by following these steps:

Sit on your mat with your legs straight. Keep your back and neck elongated.

Raise the right leg and bend it over the left one near the knee. Place the right foot on the floor next to the side of the left leg. Toes are facing front.

Only if you are able to keep both "sit bones" on the floor: Twist your left leg around, stopping at the right hip. Otherwise, remain as in step 2. Wrap the left arm around the right thigh and pull inward hugging into yourself.

Reach out behind with the right arm. Turn your head to the right.

Put your right hand on the floor behind you. Sit up straight and do not lean. If needed, use a book under your hand to remain erect. Keep your head looking over your right shoulder.

Inhaling, push your "sit bones" into the ground and stretch your spine upwards. Exhaling, increase the twist to the right in this sequence: Navel, ribs, chest, neck, and head. Breathe slowly. Gently repeat holding and increasing the twist as you breathe for up to two minutes.

Release and massage your legs. Repeat on the other side.

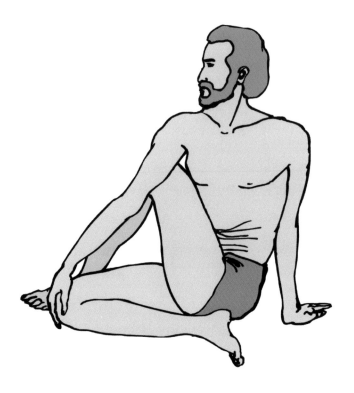

CHAPTER 16- BUTTERFLY POSE- BADHAKONASANA

The butterfly pose is a well known pose for Yoga and helps to strengthen your legs, core and even help you relax. Check out how to do it:

Sit down on a flat service. Bring the soles of your feet together until the touch, using your arms and hands if needed. Your knees should be bent at this point. Pull your heels inwards as close as possible for a better stretch, but this may take some practice depending on your flexibility. Keep your back straight and clasp your feet with your hands. Inhale, and then place a hand on each of your knees. Press on your thighs with your hands and try to stretch your legs as far as possible to the floor. Start flapping both of your legs as if you are a butterfly while clenching your feet.

Keep your breathing steady and try increase the speed of this. Bend forward after while keeping your chin and back straight. Use the elbows to press your legs and thighs down to the floor as much as possible. If you keep on practicing, you'll see a difference in how much you can press down. You should feel the stretch in your inner thighs as well as muscles in the leg area that should be relaxing. As you exhale, release posture.

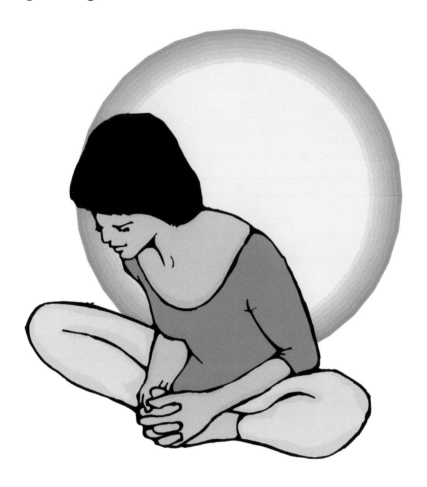

CHAPTER 17- CAT STRETCH-
MARJARIASANA

To do the cat stretch or Marjariasana, begin on all fours on your mat. Keep the hands directly beneath your shoulders, shoulder width apart with the arms perpendicular to the floor. Point the hands straight and spread the fingers apart. If your wrists hurt or you are not comfortable using your hands to support the body, you can use your elbows instead. The knees should be under your hips at hip-width apart. Make a table with your back, keep it flat. Keep your head straight and aligned with your spine, eyes should be looking at the mat.

Take a deep breath, as you breathe in, raise your chin up towards the ceiling, drop your navel towards your mat and feel tailbone lift up. Hold this position for five to ten deep breaths while relaxing the mind. After holding the position, on the next breathe exhalation, drop your chin towards your chest and arch the spine to the ceiling. The arms should be straight and the buttocks should be relaxed. Hold for five to ten breaths. The back should not be strained, go as far as your spine will allow you to without injuring yourself. As your become more flexible, you will be able to arch your back even more. After holding the position, inhale and return to the starting neutral position. You should exit the cat stretch using the child's pose.

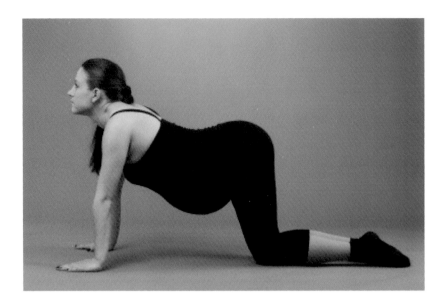

CHAPTER 18- CHILD POSE- SHISHU ASANA

Start on your hands and knees. Place the inner sides of your big toes together. Gently let your hips slide back towards your feet, keeping your knees about hip width apart. Bend forward from the hips, lowering your forehead to the floor. If this is not accessible, you can rest your head on a block (any side that is comfortable) or on your fists stacked together.

Arms can rest extended in front of you, palms up, with elbows raised off the floor. Arms can also be rested alongside your body and thighs, with palms facing upwards. Gently press your chest into your thighs as you breathe. Allow your shoulders to relax away from your ears, down to the hips and out.

To release from the pose, raise the upper body as you inhale. Try to retain the spinal lengthening you felt during the pose.

Child's pose, or Shishu Asana, is an excellent pose for resting in between vinyasas. It is also helpful for re-aligning the spine, especially the lower back. Child's pose also aids digestion, because it gently stretches the lower abdomen. The pose is also used during mediation, as it is restful and lends itself to general relaxation. It is called child's pose due to its similarity to the intuitive sleep posture of many children and infants.

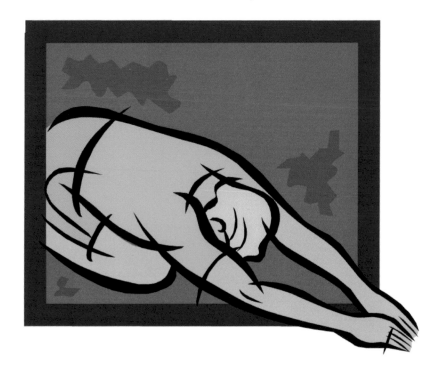

CHAPTER 19- MILL CHURNING POSE- CHAKKI CHALANASANA

To begin the Mill Churning Pose, start by sitting on your yoga mat with your back straight, chest up, and your legs stretched straight ahead, splayed apart at an angle that is not too stressful on your hips, but does gently stretch your pelvis. Flex your feet so that your toes reach back towards your chest and your heels extend forwards. Extend your arms in front of your chest and clasp your hands together, interlacing the fingers.

While keeping your legs flat on the floor, begin to move your hands around in large circles, pulling your upper body forwards as you reach out, and pushing your torso backwards as you complete the circle. Keep your arms straight and elbows locked so that your torso is forced to move with your hands. At the height of your circles you should be bent far forward, reaching out with your hands, looking forward with your head up, your back as straight as possible.

At the opposite end, you are pushing your torso backwards but being careful to keep your legs flat on the floor (at this point they will want to rise up and you may lose your balance). Go slowly and focus on stretching your arms, shoulders, hips, and hamstrings. Reverse the direction of your circles and do an equal amount in the new direction.

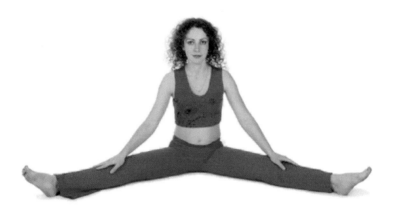

CHAPTER 20- BOW POSE- DHANURASANA

To do the Bow pose, begin by lying face down on your mat with your stomach pressed flat against the ground and your hands lying comfortably at your sides. On an exhale, bend your knees, as if trying to touch your heels to your butt while simultaneously reaching back with both hands to grab your feet by your toes or outer ankles. On an inhale, draw your heels towards the sky while pulling your shoulder and the top of your torso off the mat.

The tops of your thighs will also leave the mat. Press your shoulder blades together to lift even higher off the mat. Hold this pose for as long as you feel comfortable while controlling your breathing. Release by slowly lowering your thighs and shoulder back to your mat, and releasing your hands from your feet. Rest your arms comfortably at your side.

Beginners to Bow pose can modify the pose by starting with half Bow pose using one leg and one arm at a time until he or she can comfortably hold both hands and both feet while lifting off the mat. Additionally, a yoga strap can be used to achieve bow pose for those with less flexibility. For a more advanced modification to achieve deeper bow pose, grab opposite ankles or calves with the hand.

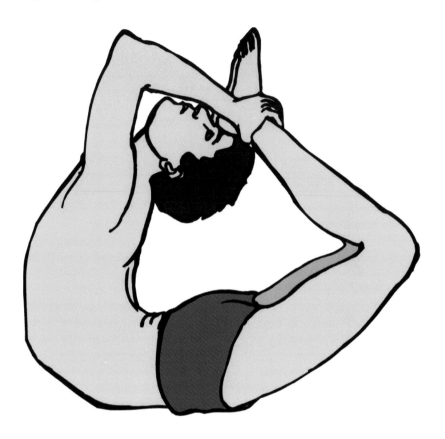

CHAPTER 21- COBRA POSE- BHUJANGASANA

The cobra pose or Bhujangsana begins with you lying on your stomach on your mat. Do not do this pose if you have any wrist or rib injuries or if you are pregnant. You should also avoid this pose if you have any abdominal injuries. While lying face down, the tops of your feet should be touching the mat. Legs are to be kept close together with the heels touching.

Place your hands palms down under your shoulders and point your elbows in towards your body, hugging the body. Inhale deeply and lift your head, chest and abdomen slowly up away from the mat. Remember to keep breathing and arch your spine slowly while keeping your navel down on your mat. If you are flexible enough, straighten your arms as you go up. Be sure you can still take full deep breaths in the position; if you find the breathing becoming shallow you are overstretching and straining the body.

Keep the shoulders relaxed and don't tighten the buttocks. If your shoulders are up too high, bend your elbows. As you continue to practice the cobra pose, you will be able to straighten your elbows while relaxing your shoulders. Hold the pose for 15 to 30 seconds making sure to continue deep, relaxed breathing. Exhale and slowly bring yourself back to the starting position.

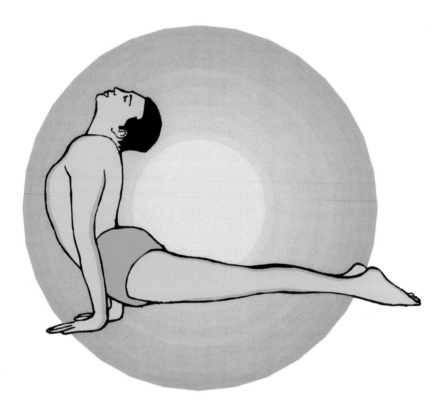

Amy Gilchrist

Chapter 22- Superman Pose- Viparita Shalabhasana

The Superman Pose or Viparita Shalabhasana, is quite easy to assume. To begin you will first need to lie completely flat on your stomach. Lightly press your toes against the floor beneath you. Your chin will also need to be lightly placed against the floor. Your right and left leg should be gently pressed together, the same goes for both feet. Your arms will need to be extended in front of you while gently resting them on the floor.

Once you are ready to begin the pose, slowly extend your arms forward as far as possible. Do not strain or attempt to overly extend. Next take a full breath and then slowly and evenly lift your legs, chest, and arms completely off the floor. Regarding your legs, do make sure that your upper thighs are also off the ground as far as is possible.

During this pose focus on steadily taking in deep breaths, and then gently exhaling them. You will also want to attempt to maintain a firm and steady balance, while simultaneously keeping your muscles as relaxed and tension free as possible. Do not stress or strain your muscles during the pose, as your goal should be to slowly and gently stretch your muscles and spine. Practice the pose daily to strengthen your balance and form.

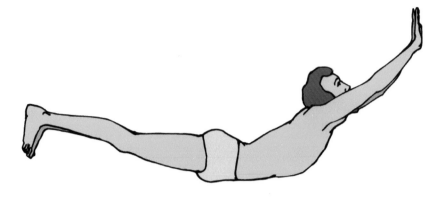

CHAPTER 23- LOCUST POSE- SHALABASANA

Lie face down on your stomach with legs together. Your forehead rests on the floor to lengthen your neck. For an alternative style, rest your chin on the floor. Place your hands flat on the floor at your sides with the elbows bent towards the ceiling. Fingers are pointing towards the toes and thumb towards the head. Advanced practitioners can grasp their hands at their back. Take two breaths in this position. Inhale. Lift both legs as high as possible off the floor while pushing down lightly with your hands. Toes should be arched towards the shins. Try to stretch all the way down to the heels.

Hold this position for 30 seconds while feeling the stretch in the lower back and legs. Don't forget to keep breathing. Exhale, release the heel stretch, and lower your legs to the floor.

For beginners, this asana can be modified by only raising one leg at a time and then repeating the pose on the other side. A soft blanket can be placed under the hip bones or thighs for comfort. To support raising the legs, place blocks under the thighs.

This asana is not recommended for people with high blood pressure or heart ailments.

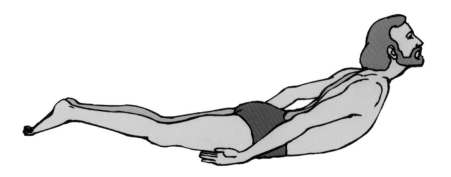

CHAPTER 24- BOAT POSE- NAUKASANA

To begin to enter Boat Pose, first start seated on your yoga mat with your arms at your sides and your legs stretched out in front of you, your chest forward, looking straight ahead. Next, rock back slightly so that your weight is balanced on your tailbone, while keeping your back straight.

Your upper half should now be at approximately a forty-five degree angle to the floor, and your feet and legs should have naturally risen up from the floor ever so slightly. Keeping your hands resting lightly on the mat for balance, begin to raise your legs. Keep your legs straight and your toes pointed; you should feel your core tensing as you fully enter the pose.

Ideally, your legs will also be at a forty-five degree angle to the floor, so that from the side you look like a perfect V-shape. However, this will take some practice. Once your legs and body are steady, lift your hands from the mat and stretch your arms out in front of you, aiming to keep them parallel with your legs. Very advanced yogis will be able to grab their toes while maintaining this pose, and so the beginner should not aim for this but rather to keep their core engaged and their balance steady. Hold this pose for at least 15 seconds at a time.

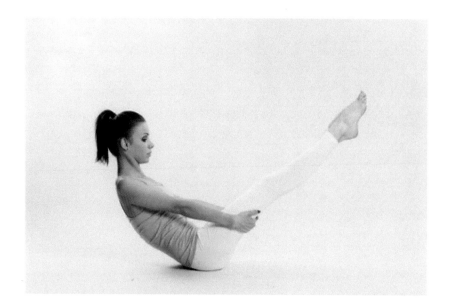

CHAPTER 25- BRIDGE POSE- SETUBANDHASANA

Yoga is a powerful and amazing way to relax your body and mind, as well as gain flexibility and strength. Check out how to do a popular yoga move, the bridge pose:

Lie on your back and bend your knees while keeping your feet around your butt. Using your feet, press down firmly onto the floor and lift your hips off of the ground. Your arms, feet, head and hands should remain on the ground. Rotate your things inward a little so that your knees do not fall to the side. If you want to go into the full position after you have mastered the first part, begin by clasping your hands underneath your back and interlace your fingers. Lift your back a little higher but remain relaxed, do not reach it to high. Now, stay in this pose and hold the position strongly. You should focus on expanding your chest, staying relaxed and scooping in your below as you exhale.

Try doing this for as long as you can hold, and then carefully get back down. As you practice, you will find that your back and hands will be able to support you in that position and you can hold the stance longer for a better pose. Release by keeping your spine straight and lowering your arms slowly.

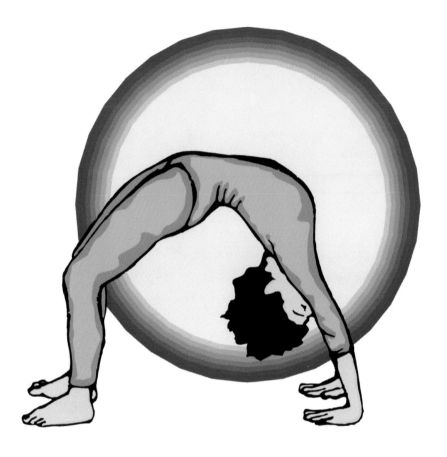

Chapter 26- Fish Pose- Matsyasana

Sit with legs crossed in Lotus Position (Padmasana). Slowly lean your torso back using your elbows and arms for support. Feel your chest opening up as you arch your back. Continue arching your torso until the crown of your head is resting lightly on the floor. You should not feel any pressure pushing it into the floor.

To release:

Slide your head down to the floor and lower your back. Breathe in as you sit up. Release your legs. Matsyasana is an advanced pose to be developed in two preliminary stages:

Stage 1 for Beginners:

Fold a towel and place it on your mat where your shoulder blades will be when you lean back. Sitting with your legs straight out in front of you, slowly lean your torso back so that your shoulders arch over the towel. Rest and breathe quietly for two minutes. Then roll over and sit up.

Stage 2 for Beginners:

Lie down with straight legs. Place your hands palms down, fingers towards toes, slightly under your buttocks. Inhale and push with the hands and lower arms to arch the back and shoulders off the floor. Tilt the head back. Hold for two minutes. Inhale while lowering torso back down, and then sit up slowly.

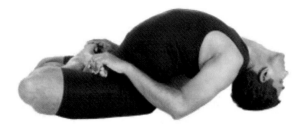

CHAPTER 27- WIND-RELIEVING POSE-PAVANAMUKTASANA

To enter Wind-Relieving Pose, begin by laying on your yoga mat facing the ceiling, your legs straight in front of you, your arms resting gently by your sides. Bend your right leg and start to bring it towards your chest, placing both hands on the leg just beneath the knee and interlacing the fingers. Keep your left leg straight on the mat, and flex your foot (toes pointing towards chest, heel extended).

Pull your right leg towards your chest as far as possible; ideally the top of your thigh will be pressed into your chest, and your knee will rest under your chin. Maintain this position until you feel your hips fully opening. When you are ready, gently and slowly straighten your right leg and return it to the mat (being careful not to stress the knee that was just bent).

Repeat this process with your left leg, taking your time and being sure to fully stretch out your pelvic area. Finally, bring both legs to the chest. You can place one hand directly under each knee, or place your knees in the crooks of your elbows and lay your forearms next to each other across both of your legs. Draw your knees towards your chin. You should feel your pelvis stretching to accommodate your rib cage as you breathe deeply. Remain here for as long as you want, then slowly return to the starting position.

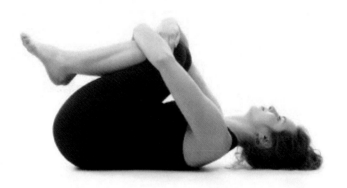

Chapter 28- Shoulder Stand-Sarvangasana

To do a correct shoulder stand you will first need to place a blanket or pad across your upper back, making sure that your neck extends beyond it. Next place your arms by your side and then assume the Plow Pose. Moving along, next you will want to lift your legs over your head using your abdominal muscles. Make sure that your toes extend towards the floor past your head. Press down against the floor while making sure to keep your back as straight as possible.

Maintaining a steady balance throughout the process is essential. Make sure to place your hands firmly by your lower back, as this will act as a balance stabilizer. While you're in this position your elbows should be resting on the blanket. Throughout the entire process make sure that your muscles are relaxed, as any tension or body stress can greatly inhibit proper balance and technique. Pay particularly close attention to the relaxation of the muscles of the neck and of those that surround your spine.

Properly exiting the shoulder stand position is very important. Using your core strength slowly lower both legs back down to the floor, making sure that your motion is controlled. It's recommended during the transition that you assume the resting Halasana pose before going back to lying completely flat again.

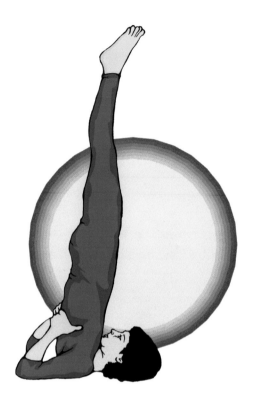

Amy Gilchrist

CHAPTER 29- PLOW POSE- HALASANA

Lie flat on the floor, with arms outstretched over head and legs together on the floor with feet flat and toes pointed up. Lift your legs up from the hips at a 45 degree angle, feet flat, toes pointed toward your head. Lift your hips off of the floor until your feet meet with the floor behind you, keeping your head flat and arms in their original position.

Lift your back so that your tailbone pushes up toward the ceiling. Straighten your back and bring your arms down until they meet behind your back. Keep your stomach tight and soften your neck so your chin does not push into your chest.

Continue holding the pose. Bring hands up behind you to support your back and continue pushing your tailbone up toward the ceiling, for up to five minutes. Inhale and slowly lift legs up toward the ceiling once again, drawing hands toward your back as you lift your feet. To further tighten the pose, walk your feet in toward your head slowly, maintaining your position in your spine, stomach and head.

Maintain the position for up to five minutes, and then release your back and put your hands flat on the floor behind you. Slowly raise your feet off of the floor, and lower your hips back to the original position and lower one leg at a time until you are flat.

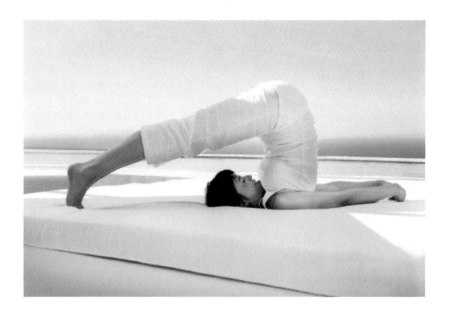

CHAPTER 30- LYING-DOWN BODY TWIST-CHAKRASANA

To enter the Lying-Down Body Twist Pose, first begin by laying on your mat facing the ceiling with your legs straight, arms relaxed by your sides. Next, bring your arms out until they are resting horizontally on the floor, perpendicular to your legs. Your arms and shoulders should be in a straight line, the palms of your hands facing the ceiling, and both of your shoulder blades flat on the floor. Bend your knees and draw your legs up until your feet are close to your buttocks. Your feet should be slightly more than hip-width apart.

Float your knees down to your left side, twisting your hips until your left leg is resting flat on the floor, your right leg on top of it. Make sure to keep your shoulders flat on the floor as well, and turn your head to the right, keeping your eye on your hand. Your right shoulder will want to rise up off the floor, but make sure to press it down to get the full effect of the stretch.

It may help to press the back of your right hand to the floor, and be conscious to maintain contact between the floor and your left knee as well. After a few minutes, float your knees up and look to the ceiling, then repeat the process on your left side.

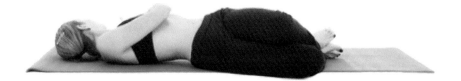

CHAPTER 31- LYING-DOWN ON SIDES- VISHNU ASANA

To do the Lying-Down on Sides Pose, start by laying on your mat facing the ceiling, with your arms by your sides. Next, roll over to your right side, using your right hand to support your head, and placing your left hand on the mat directly in front of your chest for balance. Your legs should be straight, and the left leg should be resting gently on top of the right leg.

Slowly raise your left leg into the air, keeping it on the same plane as the rest of your body (don't swing it forwards towards your chest or backwards over your buttocks). Raise your leg to the full height you are capable of; if you are flexible enough and can grab your toes with your left hand, do so now. Remain in this position for as long as it takes for your hip to feel properly stretched out.

Slowly begin to lower your leg; optionally, when it is a few inches above your right leg, you can gently draw small circles with your pointed toes, first clockwise, then counterclockwise. Maintaining control of your leg, slowly lower it further, and allow it to come to rest on top of your right leg. Return to the starting position laying on your back. Then, repeat on your left side.

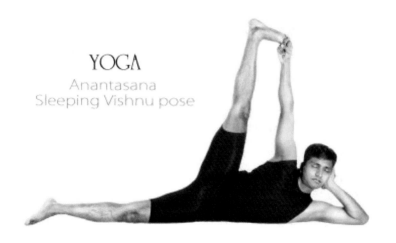

YOGA
Anantasana
Sleeping Vishnu pose

CHAPTER 32- CORPSE POSE- SHAVASANA

The Shavasana or corpse pose relaxes the body but also promotes awareness and concentration as well. Lie on your back on your mat and begin the pose by closing your eyes. Adjust your body so your limbs are symmetrical and not contorted in any way. Make sure the feet are not pointing straight up, rather relax them and have your feet fall outward to each side.

Place your arms on each side of the body. Have some distance between your hands and body. Turn your hands so your palms face the ceiling. Relax your jaw and release the tension from your face. You should feel the body sag and become heavy. Feel the body elongate and stretch away from itself. Take long deep breaths and remain aware of your surroundings. Your mind should be focused on the way the body is feeling in the pose, do not let it wander. This pose can be held for whatever amount of time you desire.

To wake the body from Shavasana, flex and your fingers and toes with your eyes still shut. You can continue to stretch your body by raising your arms over your head. Return to sitting position by using your legs to bring your body to its side. Use your arms to support yourself and return to a sitting position. Open your eyes to finish the pose.

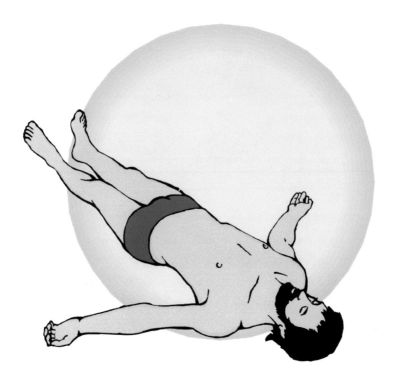